PARKINSON DISEASE DIET COOKBOOK FOR BEGINNERS

Boost Energy, Reduce Symptoms: 75 Easy Parkinson's-Friendly Recipes for Beginners

SELENA LEONARD

Copyright© 2024 [Selena Leonard]

All rights reserved. Unauthorized reproduction or distribution of this work is strictly prohibited or transmitted in any form or by any means, including photocopying, recording, or other electronic or methods, without the prior written permission of the publisher, except in the case of brief quotations embodied in critical articles and reviews.

Table of Contents

INTRODUCTION 13

EMPOWERING YOUR JOURNEY WITH PARKINSON'S THROUGH DELICIOUS FOOD 13

Understanding Parkinson's Disease and the Power of Nutrition: 13

How This Cookbook Can Help You Manage Your Symptoms and Feel Your Best: 14

A Guide to Using This Cookbook: 15

PART 1: THE ESSENTIAL PARKINSON'S DIET: 18

CHAPTER 1 19

BRAIN-BOOSTING BREAKFASTS 19

BENEFITS OF A HEALTHY BREAKFAST FOR PARKINSON'S MANAGEMENT 19

Recipes for a Brain-Boosting Start: 20

    Smoked Salmon Scramble with Berries and Walnuts (p. xx) 20

    Overnight Berry Chia Pudding with Greek Yogurt (p. xx) .. 21

    Tropical Power Bowl with Oatmeal and Fatty Fish (p. xx) .. 23

    Whole Wheat Pancakes with Nut Butter and Berries (p. xx) 24

    Frittata Fiesta with Vegetables and Eggs (p. xx) 26

CHAPTER 2 31

ENERGIZING LUNCHES AND LIGHT DINNERS 31

    The Importance of Balanced Meals for Sustained Energy 31

    Recipes for Energizing Lunches and Light Dinners: 32

        Mediterranean Chickpea Salad with Whole Wheat Pita Bread (p. xx) 32

        Tuna Salad Stuffed Avocados with a Citrus Twist (p. xx) ... 34

        Lentil Soup with Whole Grain Bread and a Side Salad (p. xx) 35

        Salmon with Roasted Vegetables and Quinoa (p. xx) 38

        Chicken Stir-Fry with Brown Rice and Mixed Greens (p. xx) 40

CHAPTER 3 43

DELICIOUS AND NOURISHING SNACKS 43

    Keeping Your Energy Levels Up Throughout the Day 43

    Recipes for Delicious and Nourishing Snacks: 44

        Trail Mix with Berries, Nuts, and Dark Chocolate (p. xx) ... 44

        Yogurt Parfait with Granola and Sliced Fruit (p. xx) 45

        Edamame Pods with a Sprinkle of Sea Salt (p. xx) 47

Hummus with Whole-Wheat Pita Bread and Sliced Vegetables (p. xx) 48

PART 2: BUILDING A PARKINSON'S-FRIENDLY DIET: 52

CHAPTER 4 53

ESSENTIAL NUTRIENTS FOR BRAIN HEALTH 53

Understanding the Role of Macronutrients and Micronutrients 53

Macronutrients: The Building Blocks.................................. 53

Micronutrients: The Power Players 54

Benefits of Specific Foods for Parkinson's Management 55

CHAPTER 5 57

FOODS TO EMBRACE AND FOODS TO LIMIT: CRAFTING A BRAIN-BOOSTING DIET.. 57

Choosing Brain-Boosting Foods and Minimizing Inflammatory Foods.. 57

Embrace These Brain-Boosting Powerhouses: 57

Minimize These Inflammatory Culprits: 59

Creating a Sustainable and Delicious Eating Pattern:........... 60

CHAPTER 6: 63

TIPS FOR EASY MEAL PLANNING WITH PARKINSON'S: .. 63

Streamlining Groceries and Meals, Adapting Recipes 63

    Streamlining Grocery Shopping: 63

    Simplifying Meal Preparation 64

    Adapting Recipes for Different Dietary Needs: 65

    Additional Tips: 66

CHAPTER 7 67

SAMPLE WEEKLY MEAL PLANS AND GROCERY LISTS: 67

    A Delicious Start to Your Healthy Journey 67

    Sample Weekly Meal Plan 1: 67

    Sunday: 67

    Breakfast (Greek Yogurt Parfait with Berries, Granola, and Honey): 67

    Lunch 69

    (Tuna Salad Sandwich on Whole-Wheat Bread with Lettuce, Tomato, and Avocado Slices, Side Salad with Mixed Greens and Vinaigrette Dressing): 69

    Dinner (Salmon with Roasted Vegetables and Quinoa): 70

    Snacks: 71

    Sample Weekly Meal Plan 2 (Vegetarian Option): 71

Sunday: 71

   Breakfast (Chia Pudding with Almond Milk, Berries, and Chia Seeds): 71

Monday: 72

   Breakfast (Scrambled Eggs with Spinach and Whole-Wheat Toast): 72

   Lunch 73

   (Leftover Salmon with a Side of Brown Rice and Steamed Green Beans): 73

   Dinner (Chicken Stir-Fry with Brown Rice and Mixed Vegetables): 74

   Snacks: 76

Tuesday: 76

   Breakfast (Oatmeal with Chopped Walnuts, Blueberries, and a Sprinkle of Cinnamon): 76

   Lunch 77

   (Lentil Soup with a Side Salad and Whole-Wheat Bread): .. 77

   Dinner 78

   (Turkey Chili with Whole-Wheat Cornbread (optional)): 78

   Snacks: 79

Wednesday: 79

    Breakfast 79

    (Smoothie made with Greek Yogurt, Berries, Spinach, and a Splash of Almond Milk): 79

    Lunch (Chickpea Salad Sandwich on Whole-Wheat Bread with Lettuce, Tomato, and Cucumber): 80

    Dinner (Baked Cod with Roasted Sweet Potato and Steamed Asparagus): 82

PART 3: LIVING A VIBRANT LIFE WITH PARKINSON'S: .. 84

CHAPTER 8: 85

ADDITIONAL LIFESTYLE TIPS FOR OPTIMAL HEALTH: . 85

    Exercise, Sleep, and Stress Management................................. 85

        The Power of Exercise: 85

        Finding the Right Exercise for You: 86

        Tips for Better Sleep: 87

        Stress Management for Parkinson's: 88

        Relaxation Techniques: 88

CHAPTER 9 91

COOKING WITH PARKINSON'S 91

Helpful Adaptations for Independence in the Kitchen 91

Kitchen Techniques for Easier Meal Preparation: 92

Maintaining Independence in the Kitchen: 93

BONUS Parkinson's-Friendly Recipes for Beginners: 97

Delicious and Easy Meals 97

Breakfast 97

Power Berry Oatmeal (Serves 1 97

Scrambled Eggs with Spinach and Tomatoes (Serves 1) 98

Greek Yogurt Parfait with Berries and Granola (Serves 1) 100

Chia Pudding with Berries and Almond Milk (Serves 1) ... 101

Whole-Wheat Toast with Sliced Avocado and Eggs (Serves 1) 102

Smoothie with Greek Yogurt, Berries, and Spinach (Serves 1) 103

Banana Pancakes with Walnuts (Serves 1) 104

Scrambled Tofu with Vegetables (Serves 1) 105

Overnight Oats with Berries and Chia Seeds (Serves 1) 106

Cottage Cheese with Sliced Fruit and Honey (Serves 1) 107

Lunch 108

Salmon with Roasted Vegetables (Serves 1) 108

Greek Yogurt Chicken Salad Sandwich (Serves 1) 109

Tuna Salad with Whole-Wheat Crackers (Serves 1) 110

Egg Salad Sandwich with Avocado (Serves 1).................... 112

Lentil Soup with Whole-Wheat Bread (Serves 1) 113

Chicken and Veggie Wrap (Serves 1)................................... 114

Berry Salad with Walnuts and Yogurt Dressing (Serves.... 115

Open-Faced Turkey and Avocado Sandwich (Serves 1).... 116

Cottage Cheese with Fruit and Granola (Serves 1)............. 117

Egg Salad Lettuce Wraps (Serves.. 118

Dinner 119

Baked Salmon with Roasted Vegetables and Quinoa (Serves 1) 119

Scrambled Eggs with Spinach, Tomatoes, and Whole-Wheat Toast (Serves 1) 121

Greek Yogurt Chicken Bowl with Berries (Serves 1) 122

Turkey Meatloaf with Roasted Vegetables (Serves 1) 123

Whole-Wheat Pasta with Shrimp and Vegetables (Serves 1) 125

Walnut-Crusted Salmon with Roasted Brussels Sprouts (Serves 1) 126

Egg Drop Soup with Vegetables (Serves 1) 127

Cottage Cheese with Fruit and Granola 129

Snacks 130

Fruit and Nut Mix (Serves 1) 130

Greek Yogurt with Chia Seeds and Honey (Serves 1) 131

Hard-Boiled Eggs with Sliced Vegetables (Serves 1) 132

Trail Mix (Serves 1) 132

Cottage Cheese with Pineapple and Sliced Almonds (Serves 1) 133

Edamame Pods with Sea Salt (Serves 1) 134

Apple Slices with Almond Butter (Serves 1) 135

Whole-Wheat Crackers with Hummus and Vegetables (Serves 1) 136

Cottage Cheese Smoothie (Serves 1) 137

Roasted Chickpeas with Spices (Serves 1) 138

CONCLUSION 141

EMBRACING DELICIOUS AND NUTRITIOUS EATING WITH PARKINSON'S DISEASE 141

INTRODUCTION

EMPOWERING YOUR JOURNEY WITH PARKINSON'S THROUGH DELICIOUS FOOD

Parkinson's disease can present a daily challenge, but you are not alone in this journey. Did you know that what you eat can play a significant role in managing your symptoms and improving your overall well-being? This cookbook is designed to be your empowering companion, offering a delicious and practical approach to navigating the world of Parkinson's-friendly nutrition.

Understanding Parkinson's Disease and the Power of Nutrition:

Parkinson's disease is a neurological condition that affects the central nervous system, leading to symptoms like tremors, stiffness, and difficulty with balance. While there is no cure, a growing body of research suggests that a well-balanced diet rich in specific nutrients can significantly improve your quality of life. This includes:

- **Supporting Brain Health:** Certain foods provide essential nutrients that nourish brain cells and may help protect them from damage associated with Parkinson's.
- **Managing Inflammation:** Chronic inflammation is linked to Parkinson's progression. This cookbook focuses on anti-inflammatory ingredients to help mitigate its effects.
- **Boosting Energy Levels:** Fatigue is a common symptom. We'll explore recipes that provide sustained energy throughout the day.
- **Optimizing Gut Health:** A healthy gut microbiome is crucial for overall well-being and may influence Parkinson's symptoms. We'll incorporate gut-friendly ingredients.

How This Cookbook Can Help You Manage Your Symptoms and Feel Your Best:

This book goes beyond just recipes. It's a comprehensive guide designed to empower you to take control of your diet and feel your best with Parkinson's. Here's what you can expect:

- **75 Easy and Delicious Recipes:** We've curated a collection of simple yet flavorful recipes that are packed with brain-boosting nutrients. They are beginner-friendly and require minimal prep time.
- **Focus on Symptom Management:** Each recipe is chosen with specific Parkinson's symptoms in mind, making it easier to find meals that target your individual needs.
- **Nutritional Information:** All recipes include clear nutritional breakdowns, allowing you to make informed choices that align with your dietary goals.
- **Dietary Tips & Modifications:** We provide guidance for adapting recipes to accommodate different dietary restrictions or preferences.
- **Meal Planning Strategies:** Learn valuable tips for planning balanced and delicious meals throughout the week, saving you time and stress.

A Guide to Using This Cookbook:

To make navigating this cookbook a breeze, we've included some helpful features:

- **Symbols:** Recipes are categorized with icons to indicate their focus (e.g., breakfast, energizing lunch, gut-friendly).

- **Tips:** Scattered throughout the book are essential tips for maximizing the benefits of your meals and navigating the kitchen with Parkinson's.
- **Meal Planning Section:** A dedicated section offers templates and strategies for creating personalized weekly meal plans that fit your needs.

This cookbook is more than just a collection of recipes; it's a starting point for a healthier and more empowered journey with Parkinson's. We believe that delicious food can be a powerful tool in managing your symptoms and living a vibrant life. Let's get started on this culinary adventure together!

PART 1: THE ESSENTIAL PARKINSON'S DIET:

CHAPTER 1

BRAIN-BOOSTING BREAKFASTS

BENEFITS OF A HEALTHY BREAKFAST FOR PARKINSON'S MANAGEMENT

Skipping breakfast can worsen Parkinson's symptoms such as fatigue and tremors. A healthy breakfast sets the tone for the day by providing sustained energy, improving focus, and promoting overall well-being. Here's how:

- **Boosts Energy Levels:** Choosing complex carbohydrates and healthy fats provides a slow and steady release of energy, helping you feel energized throughout the morning.
- **Supports Brain Function:** Essential nutrients like Omega-3 fatty acids, antioxidants, and B vitamins found in a balanced breakfast are crucial for brain health and may play a role in protecting brain cells.
- **Improves Mood and Focus:** A healthy breakfast can help regulate blood sugar levels, contributing to better mood,

improved cognitive function, and sharper focus throughout the day.

- **Reduces Inflammation:** Certain breakfast foods are rich in anti-inflammatory properties, which may help manage chronic inflammation associated with Parkinson's.

Recipes for a Brain-Boosting Start:

This chapter offers a variety of delicious and easy-to-prepare breakfast options packed with brain-boosting nutrients:

Smoked Salmon Scramble with Berries and Walnuts (p. xx)

Ingredients:

- 2 large eggs
- 1 tablespoon unsweetened almond milk
- 1/4 cup chopped spinach or kale
- 2 ounces smoked salmon, flaked
- 1/2 cup fresh berries (blueberries, raspberries)
- 1/4 cup chopped walnuts

Instructions:

- In a bowl, whisk together eggs and almond milk.
- Heat a non-stick pan over medium heat. Spray with cooking spray (optional).

- Add the spinach or kale and cook until wilted, about 1 minute.
- Pour in the egg mixture and scramble with a spatula until cooked through, approximately 3-4 minutes.
- Top with smoked salmon, berries, and walnuts.

Nutritional Facts (per serving):

- Calories: 350
- Protein: 20g
- Fat: 18g
- Carbohydrates: 20g
- Fiber: 3g

Tips:

- Feel free to use low-fat feta cheese instead of smoked salmon for a variation.
- For extra creaminess, stir in a tablespoon of plain full-fat Greek yogurt after scrambling the eggs.
- If chopping vegetables is a challenge, use pre-washed and chopped spinach or kale.

Overnight Berry Chia Pudding with Greek Yogurt (p. xx)

Ingredients:

- 1/4 cup chia seeds
- 1 cup unsweetened almond milk or coconut milk
- 1 tablespoon honey or maple syrup (optional)
- 1/2 teaspoon vanilla extract
- 1/2 cup plain Greek yogurt
- 1/2 cup fresh berries (blueberries, raspberries)
- Sliced almonds (optional)

Instructions:

- In a jar or container with a lid, combine chia seeds, milk, honey (if using), and vanilla extract.
- Stir well, cover, and refrigerate overnight.
- In the morning, top with Greek yogurt, fresh berries, and sliced almonds (optional).

Nutritional Facts (per serving):

- Calories: 300
- Protein: 15g
- Fat: 12g
- Carbohydrates: 30g
- Fiber: 8g

Tips:

- For a thicker pudding, use 1/3 cup chia seeds.
- Substitute honey or maple syrup with a mashed banana for added sweetness and natural sugars.
- Explore different flavor options by adding a sprinkle of cinnamon, nutmeg, or cocoa powder to the chia seed mixture.

Tropical Power Bowl with Oatmeal and Fatty Fish (p. xx)

Ingredients:

- 1/2 cup rolled oats
- 1 cup water or unsweetened plant-based milk
- 3 ounces poached or grilled salmon or tuna (flaked)
- 1/2 cup chopped mango
- 1/2 cup chopped pineapple
- 1 tablespoon chia seeds
- 1/4 cup low-sugar yogurt or coconut milk (optional)

Instructions:

- In a saucepan, bring water or milk to a boil. Add rolled oats and cook on low heat for 5 minutes, or until desired consistency is reached.
- While the oatmeal cooks, poach or grill the fish according to package instructions. Flake the cooked fish.

- In a bowl, combine cooked oatmeal, flaked fish, chopped mango, chopped pineapple, and chia seeds.
- Top with a dollop of low-sugar yogurt or coconut milk (optional).

Nutritional Facts (per serving):

- Calories: 400
- Protein: 25g
- Fat: 15g
- Carbohydrates: 40g
- Fiber: 5g

Tips:

- This recipe is easily customizable. Use other berries or chopped fruits like papaya instead of mango and pineapple.
- If poaching or grilling fish is challenging, consider using canned tuna packed in water. Drain well and flake before adding to the bowl.
- For extra protein and creaminess, add a scoop of protein powder to the cooked oatmeal while it's still hot.

Whole Wheat Pancakes with Nut Butter and Berries (p. xx)

Ingredients:

- 1 cup whole wheat flour
- 1 teaspoon baking powder
- 1/4 teaspoon salt
- 1 cup unsweetened almond milk or low-fat milk
- 1 egg
- 1 tablespoon melted coconut oil or vegetable oil
- 1/4 cup of your favorite nut butter (almond, peanut, cashew)
- 1/2 cup fresh berries (blueberries, raspberries)

Instructions:

- In a medium bowl, whisk together flour, baking powder, and salt.
- In a separate bowl, whisk together almond milk, egg, and melted oil.
- Add the wet ingredients to the dry ingredients and mix until just combined (a few lumps are okay).
- Preheat a lightly greased griddle or pan over medium heat.
- Pour 1/4 cup batter for each pancake. Cook for 2-3 minutes per side, or until golden brown and cooked through.
- Spread each pancake with your favorite nut butter and top with fresh berries.

Nutritional Facts (per serving - 2 pancakes):

- Calories: 350
- Protein: 15g
- Fat: 12g
- Carbohydrates: 40g
- Fiber: 5g

Tips:

- Make a big batch of pancake batter on the weekend and store leftover batter in the refrigerator for up to 2 days for quick weekday breakfasts.
- If flipping pancakes is challenging, consider using a pancake mold for perfectly shaped pancakes.
- Experiment with different nut butters for variety. Opt for natural nut butters with no added sugar for a healthier choice.

Frittata Fiesta with Vegetables and Eggs (p. xx)

Ingredients:

- 1 tablespoon olive oil
- 1/2 cup chopped bell pepper (any color)
- 1/2 cup chopped onion

- 1/2 cup chopped spinach or kale
- 4 large eggs, beaten
- 1/4 cup crumbled feta cheese (optional)
- 1/4 cup shredded low-fat mozzarella cheese (optional)
- Salt and pepper to taste

Instructions:

- Preheat oven to 375°F (190°C).
- Heat olive oil in an oven-safe skillet over medium heat. Add bell pepper and onion, and cook until softened, about 5 minutes.
- Add spinach or kale and cook until wilted, about 1 minute.
- Pour in the beaten eggs and stir gently to combine with the vegetables.
- Sprinkle with feta cheese and mozzarella cheese (if using).
- Bake for 15-20 minutes, or until the eggs are set and the top is golden brown.
- Season with salt and pepper to taste.

Nutritional Facts (per serving - 1/4 of the frittata):

- Calories: 250
- Protein: 15g

- Fat: 12g
- Carbohydrates: 5g
- Fiber: 2g

Tips:

- This recipe is a great way to use up leftover vegetables. Feel free to add other chopped vegetables like mushrooms, zucchini, or broccoli.
- For a vegetarian option, omit the feta cheese.
- Let the frittata cool slightly before cutting into wedges for easier handling.

CHAPTER 2

ENERGIZING LUNCHES AND LIGHT DINNERS

The Importance of Balanced Meals for Sustained Energy

Maintaining energy levels throughout the day is crucial for managing Parkinson's symptoms. Balanced lunches and light dinners provide sustained energy without feeling heavy or sluggish. Here's how:

- **Choosing Complex Carbohydrates:** Complex carbs like whole grains, legumes, and some vegetables offer a slow and steady release of energy, helping you avoid afternoon crashes.

- **Including Protein:** Protein promotes satiety and helps regulate blood sugar, which can contribute to sustained energy levels.

- **Healthy Fats:** Including healthy fats from sources like avocados, nuts, and olive oil provides satiety and keeps you feeling fuller for longer.
- **Fiber:** Fiber slows down digestion, promoting steadier blood sugar levels and preventing energy dips.

Recipes for Energizing Lunches and Light Dinners:

This chapter offers a variety of delicious and easy-to-prepare lunch and light dinner options that are packed with the nutrients you need to stay energized:

Mediterranean Chickpea Salad with Whole Wheat Pita Bread (p. xx)

Ingredients:

- 1 (15 oz) can chickpeas, drained and rinsed
- 1/2 cucumber, diced (peeled if desired)
- 1/2 red bell pepper, diced
- 1/2 red onion, finely chopped
- 2 tablespoons olive oil
- 1 1/2 tablespoons balsamic vinegar
- 1/2 teaspoon dried oregano

- 1/4 teaspoon fresh ground pepper
- 1/4 cup chopped fresh parsley
- 2-3 whole wheat pita breads, cut in half

Instructions:

- In a large bowl, combine chickpeas, cucumber, bell pepper, and red onion.
- In a small bowl, whisk together olive oil, balsamic vinegar, oregano, and pepper.
- Pour the dressing over the chickpea mixture and toss to coat.
- Stir in chopped parsley.
- Serve the chickpea salad on whole wheat pita bread halves.

Nutritional Facts (per serving - 1 pita bread with salad):

- Calories: 300
- Protein: 10g
- Fat: 10g
- Carbohydrates: 35g
- Fiber: 5g

Tips:

- Feel free to add other chopped vegetables like chopped tomatoes or kalamata olives for extra flavor and texture.
- If chopping vegetables is a challenge, purchase pre-washed and chopped vegetables.
- To make this recipe ahead of time, store the chickpea salad in an airtight container in the refrigerator for up to 3 days.

Tuna Salad Stuffed Avocados with a Citrus Twist (p. xx)

Ingredients:

- 2 ripe avocados, halved and pitted
- 5 oz canned tuna packed in water, drained and flaked
- 1/4 cup chopped celery
- 1 tablespoon chopped red onion
- 1 tablespoon chopped fresh parsley
- 2 tablespoons lemon juice
- 1 tablespoon olive oil
- Salt and pepper to taste

Instructions:

- Scoop out a small amount of avocado flesh from each half to create a well for the filling.
- In a bowl, combine flaked tuna, celery, red onion, parsley, lemon juice, and olive oil.

- Season with salt and pepper to taste.
- Gently stuff the avocado halves with the tuna salad mixture.
- Serve immediately.

Nutritional Facts (per serving - 1 stuffed avocado):

- Calories: 350
- Protein: 20g
- Fat: 20g
- Carbohydrates: 10g
- Fiber: 5g

Tips:

- Choose ripe avocados that yield slightly to gentle pressure.
- If you don't have fresh parsley, you can substitute with 1/2 teaspoon dried parsley.
- For a spicier kick, add a pinch of cayenne pepper to the tuna salad mixture.

Lentil Soup with Whole Grain Bread and a Side Salad (p. xx)

Ingredients:

- 1 tablespoon olive oil
- 1 onion, chopped

- 2 carrots, chopped
- 2 celery stalks, chopped
- 2 cloves garlic, minced
- 1 cup green lentils, rinsed
- 4 cups vegetable broth
- 1 (14.5 oz) can diced tomatoes, undrained
- 1 teaspoon dried thyme
- 1/2 teaspoon dried oregano
- Salt and pepper to taste
- 2 slices whole grain bread, toasted
- Side salad (mixed greens, cherry tomatoes, vinaigrette dressing)

Instructions:

- Heat olive oil in a large pot over medium heat.
- Add onion, carrots, and celery. Sauté for 5 minutes, or until softened.
- Add garlic and cook for an additional minute, until fragrant.
- Stir in lentils, vegetable broth, diced tomatoes, thyme, and oregano.

- Bring to a boil, then reduce heat and simmer for 20-25 minutes, or until lentils are tender.
- Season with salt and pepper to taste.
- While the soup simmers, prepare your side salad with mixed greens, cherry tomatoes, and vinaigrette dressing.
- Serve the lentil soup hot with toasted whole-grain bread and a side salad.

Nutritional Facts (per serving - 1 cup soup, 2 slices bread, side salad):

- Calories: 450
- Protein: 18g
- Fat: 15g
- Carbohydrates: 50g
- Fiber: 10g

Tips:

- This soup is easily customizable. Add other chopped vegetables like zucchini, spinach, or potatoes for extra variety.
- Leftover lentil soup can be stored in an airtight container in the refrigerator for up to 3 days or frozen for longer storage.

- If chopping vegetables is a challenge, purchase pre-washed and chopped vegetables.

Salmon with Roasted Vegetables and Quinoa (p. xx)

Ingredients:

- 4 oz salmon fillet
- 1 tablespoon olive oil
- 1/2 red onion, chopped
- 1/2 red bell pepper, chopped
- 1 cup broccoli florets
- 1/2 cup quinoa, rinsed
- 1 cup vegetable broth
- 1/4 cup chopped fresh parsley
- Salt and pepper to taste

Instructions:

- Preheat oven to 400°F (200°C).
- Toss salmon with 1/2 tablespoon olive oil, salt, and pepper.
- In a separate bowl, toss chopped onion, bell pepper, and broccoli florets with the remaining 1/2 tablespoon olive oil, salt, and pepper.
- Spread the vegetables on a baking sheet. Place the salmon on top of the vegetables.

- Roast for 15-20 minutes, or until the salmon is cooked through and the vegetables are tender-crisp.
- While the salmon and vegetables roast, cook the quinoa according to package instructions.
- To serve, spoon cooked quinoa on a plate. Top with roasted vegetables and salmon.
- Garnish with chopped fresh parsley.

Nutritional Facts (per serving):

- Calories: 450
- Protein: 30g
- Fat: 15g
- Carbohydrates: 35g
- Fiber: 5g

Tips:

- Salmon can be substituted with other types of fish like cod, tilapia, or halibut.
- Quinoa can be cooked in advance and stored in an airtight container in the refrigerator for up to 5 days.
- For added flavor, marinate the salmon in your favorite marinade for 30 minutes before baking.

Chicken Stir-Fry with Brown Rice and Mixed Greens (p. xx)

Ingredients:

- 1 tablespoon olive oil
- 1 boneless, skinless chicken breast, thinly sliced
- 1/2 cup chopped onion
- 1/2 cup chopped bell pepper (any color)
- 1/2 cup broccoli florets
- 1/4 cup chopped carrots
- 1 cup cooked brown rice
- 1/4 cup low-sodium soy sauce
- 1 tablespoon honey
- 1 tablespoon cornstarch
- 1 tablespoon sriracha (optional)
- Mixed greens salad with vinaigrette dressing

Instructions:

- In a small bowl, whisk together soy sauce, honey, cornstarch, and sriracha (if using).
- Heat olive oil in a large skillet or wok over medium-high heat.
- Add chicken and cook until browned and cooked through, about 5 minutes.

- Add onion, bell pepper, broccoli, and carrots. Stir-fry for 3-4 minutes, or until vegetables are tender-crisp.
- Pour the soy sauce mixture into the pan and stir to coat the chicken and vegetables.
- Cook for an additional minute, or until the sauce thickens slightly.
- Serve the stir-fry over cooked brown rice with a side salad of mixed greens with vinaigrette dressing.

Nutritional Facts (per serving):

- Calories: 400
- Protein: 30g
- Fat: 10g
- Carbohydrates: 40g
- Fiber: 5g

Tips:

- This recipe is easily customizable. Feel free to add other chopped vegetables like snow peas, zucchini, or mushrooms.
- Pre-cook chicken or brown rice in advance to save time during preparation. Cooked chicken and brown rice can be

stored in an airtight container in the refrigerator for up to 3 days.
- Adjust the amount of sriracha to your desired spice level.
- For a vegetarian option, omit the chicken and add an extra 1/2 cup of tofu, cubed and pan-fried before adding the vegetables.

CHAPTER 3

DELICIOUS AND NOURISHING SNACKS

Keeping Your Energy Levels Up Throughout the Day

Maintaining stable energy levels throughout the day is crucial for managing Parkinson's symptoms. Choosing healthy snacks between meals can help prevent blood sugar crashes and keep you feeling energized. Here's why healthy snacking matters:

- ✓ **Provides Sustained Energy:** Healthy snacks provide a steady stream of energy by including complex carbohydrates, protein, and healthy fats. This helps avoid the afternoon slump and prevents overeating at mealtimes.
- ✓ **Manages Blood Sugar Levels:** Choosing snacks with a balance of carbohydrates, protein, and fiber helps regulate

blood sugar levels, contributing to better mood, focus, and energy.
- ✓ **Boosts Nutrient Intake:** Snacking on nutritious options ensures you're meeting your daily needs for essential vitamins, minerals, and antioxidants which can benefit brain health and overall well-being.

Recipes for Delicious and Nourishing Snacks:

This chapter offers a variety of quick and easy snack ideas that are packed with the nutrients you need to stay energized:

Trail Mix with Berries, Nuts, and Dark Chocolate (p. xx)

Ingredients:

- 1/2 cup unsalted raw almonds
- 1/4 cup dried cranberries
- 1/4 cup dried blueberries
- 1/4 cup dark chocolate chips (at least 70% cacao)
- 1/4 cup pumpkin seeds

Instructions:

- In a medium bowl, combine almonds, cranberries, blueberries, dark chocolate chips, and pumpkin seeds.

- Toss to coat evenly.
- Store in an airtight container for up to a week.

Nutritional Facts (per 1/4 cup serving):

- Calories: 200
- Protein: 5g
- Fat: 12g
- Carbohydrates: 15g
- Fiber: 3g

Tips:

- Feel free to customize this recipe to your preferences. Substitute other nuts like cashews or walnuts, or dried fruit like cherries or apricots.
- Opt for unsalted or dry-roasted nuts for a lower sodium option.
- Choose dark chocolate with a higher cacao content for added antioxidants.

Yogurt Parfait with Granola and Sliced Fruit (p. xx)

Ingredients:

- 1 cup plain Greek yogurt
- 1/4 cup granola (choose a low-sugar variety)

- 1/2 cup sliced fresh fruit (berries, banana, mango)
- 1 tablespoon honey or maple syrup (optional)

Instructions:

- In a small parfait glass or bowl, layer 1/3 cup of Greek yogurt, followed by 1/4 cup granola, and 1/3 cup sliced fruit.
- Repeat layers one more time, ending with fruit on top.
- Drizzle with honey or maple syrup (optional).

Nutritional Facts (per serving):

- Calories: 300
- Protein: 15g
- Fat: 10g
- Carbohydrates: 35g
- Fiber: 5g

Tips:

- Use pre-cut frozen fruit for a quick and convenient option. Thaw slightly before layering in the parfait.
- If desired, add a sprinkle of chia seeds or chopped nuts for extra protein and healthy fats.

- Make a batch of parfaits ahead of time and store them in the refrigerator overnight for a grab-and-go breakfast or snack.

Edamame Pods with a Sprinkle of Sea Salt (p. xx)

Ingredients:

- 1 cup frozen shelled edamame
- Sea salt, to taste

Instructions:

- Bring a pot of water to a boil.
- Add frozen edamame and cook for 3-5 minutes, or according to package instructions.
- Drain the edamame and rinse with cold water to stop the cooking process.
- Sprinkle with sea salt to taste.

Nutritional Facts (per 1 cup serving):

- Calories: 180
- Protein: 17g
- Fat: 8g
- Carbohydrates: 20g
- Fiber: 8g

Tips:

- Look for frozen edamame pods that are already shelled for added convenience.
- For extra flavor, sprinkle the cooked edamame with a pinch of cayenne pepper or chili flakes.
- Edamame pods can be enjoyed warm or cold.

Hummus with Whole-Wheat Pita Bread and Sliced Vegetables (p. xx)

Ingredients:

- 1 cup hummus (choose a variety made with olive oil)
- 2 whole-wheat pita breads, cut into wedges
- 1 cup assorted sliced vegetables (baby carrots, cucumber slices, bell pepper strips)

Instructions:

- Spread a generous amount of hummus on whole-wheat pita wedges.
- Arrange sliced vegetables on a plate for dipping.

Nutritional Facts (per serving - 1/2 cup hummus, 2 pita wedges, and assorted vegetables):

- Calories: 350
- Protein: 10g
- Fat: 15g
- Carbohydrates: 35g
- Fiber: 5g

Tips:

- Pre-cut vegetables save time and make this a more convenient snack option.
- Experiment with different hummus flavors like roasted red pepper hummus or black bean hummus for variety.
- For extra protein, add a sprinkle of crumbled feta cheese or a dollop of plain Greek yogurt on top of the hummus.

5. Cottage Cheese with Berries and a Drizzle of Honey (p. xx)

Ingredients:

- 1/2 cup low-fat cottage cheese
- 1/2 cup fresh berries (blueberries, raspberries, strawberries)
- 1 tablespoon honey (optional)

Instructions:

- In a bowl, combine cottage cheese and fresh berries.
- Drizzle with honey (optional).

Nutritional Facts (per serving):

- Calories: 150
- Protein: 15g
- Fat: 2g
- Carbohydrates: 15g
- Fiber: 1g

Tips:

- Substitute sliced peaches, mangoes, or pears for berries for a seasonal twist.
- For extra flavor, stir in a teaspoon of vanilla extract or almond extract to the cottage cheese.
- Cottage cheese is a great source of calcium, which is important for bone health.

PART 2: BUILDING A PARKINSON'S-FRIENDLY DIET:

CHAPTER 4

ESSENTIAL NUTRIENTS FOR BRAIN HEALTH

Understanding the Role of Macronutrients and Micronutrients

The health of your brain is paramount in managing Parkinson's disease. This chapter delves into the essential nutrients that play a crucial role in brain function and explores how specific foods can be beneficial for Parkinson's management.

Macronutrients: The Building Blocks

Macronutrients are the major sources of energy for your body. They include:

- ✓ **Carbohydrates:** Complex carbohydrates, found in whole grains, fruits, and vegetables, provide sustained energy for brain function. Simple carbohydrates, like those found in sugary drinks and processed foods, should be limited as they can cause blood sugar spikes and crashes.
- ✓ **Proteins:** Proteins are the building blocks of cells, including brain cells. They are essential for

neurotransmitter production, which plays a role in movement, memory, and mood. Lean protein sources like fish, poultry, beans, and lentils are recommended.

- ✓ **Healthy Fats:** Healthy fats, found in sources like avocados, nuts, seeds, and olive oil, are crucial for brain cell health and function. They also aid in the absorption of certain vitamins. Limit unhealthy fats like saturated and trans fats found in processed foods and red meat.

Micronutrients: The Power Players

Micronutrients, including vitamins, minerals, and antioxidants, are essential for overall health and brain function. Here are some key micronutrients to focus on:

- ✓ **B Vitamins:** B vitamins, particularly B12, B6, and folate, are crucial for nerve function and neurotransmitter production. They are found in lean protein sources, whole grains, and leafy green vegetables.
- ✓ **Vitamin D:** Vitamin D plays a role in brain cell health and may have neuroprotective benefits. Sources include fatty fish, eggs, and fortified foods. Sunlight exposure also helps your body produce vitamin D.

- ✓ **Vitamin E:** Vitamin E is an antioxidant that may help protect brain cells from damage. Nuts, seeds, and olive oil are good sources.
- ✓ **Omega-3 Fatty Acids:** Omega-3 fatty acids, particularly DHA, are essential for brain function and may have anti-inflammatory properties. Fatty fish like salmon, tuna, and sardines are rich in omega-3s.
- ✓ **Antioxidants:** Antioxidants help fight free radicals that can damage brain cells. Fruits, vegetables, and spices are all rich in antioxidants.

Benefits of Specific Foods for Parkinson's Management

While there is no single food that can cure Parkinson's, incorporating a variety of nutrient-rich foods into your diet can be beneficial for managing symptoms:

- ✓ **Fruits and Vegetables:** Rich in antioxidants, vitamins, and fiber, fruits and vegetables help protect brain cells and may reduce inflammation. Choose a variety of colors to ensure a broad range of nutrients.
- ✓ **Berries:** Berries are packed with antioxidants that may help protect brain cells from damage. Blueberries, strawberries, and raspberries are all excellent choices.

- ✓ **Fatty Fish:** Fatty fish are rich in omega-3 fatty acids, which may have neuroprotective benefits and may help improve cognitive function. Aim for 2-3 servings of fatty fish per week.
- ✓ **Nuts and Seeds:** Nuts and seeds are a good source of healthy fats, protein, fiber, and vitamin E. They can also help with feelings of satiety and manage blood sugar levels.
- ✓ **Legumes:** Beans, lentils, and chickpeas are a good source of plant-based protein, fiber, and B vitamins. They are a versatile and affordable addition to your diet.
- ✓ **Green Tea:** Green tea contains antioxidants that may have neuroprotective properties. Enjoy green tea in moderation, limiting added sugars.

A balanced and varied diet is essential for overall health and Parkinson's management.

Focus on incorporating these nutrient-rich foods into your meals and snacks throughout the day.

CHAPTER 5

FOODS TO EMBRACE AND FOODS TO LIMIT: CRAFTING A BRAIN-BOOSTING DIET

Choosing Brain-Boosting Foods and Minimizing Inflammatory Foods

Parkinson's disease is a complex neurological condition. While there's no single dietary cure, research suggests that certain foods can support brain health and potentially alleviate symptoms, while others may contribute to inflammation and worsen symptoms. This chapter delves into the concept of "brain-boosting" foods and those to limit for a sustainable and delicious eating pattern in Parkinson's management.

Embrace These Brain-Boosting Powerhouses:

1. Colorful Fruits and Vegetables: These vibrant gems are loaded with antioxidants, vitamins, minerals, and fiber. Antioxidants help combat free radicals, which can damage brain cells. Fruits and vegetables also provide essential micronutrients for neurotransmitter production and overall brain function. **Focus on:**

- **Berries:** Blueberries, strawberries, raspberries, and cherries are antioxidant powerhouses rich in anthocyanins, which may have neuroprotective benefits.
- **Leafy Greens:** Kale, spinach, collard greens, and Swiss chard are packed with vitamins K and E, folate, and carotenoids, all crucial for brain health.
- **Cruciferous Vegetables:** Broccoli, cauliflower, Brussels sprouts, and cabbage contain sulforaphane, which may have anti-inflammatory properties.

2. Fatty Fish: Salmon, tuna, sardines, mackerel, and herring are rich in omega-3 fatty acids, particularly DHA. Omega-3s play a vital role in brain cell health and may improve cognitive function. Aim for 2-3 servings of fatty fish per week.

3. Nuts and Seeds: Walnuts, almonds, cashews, chia seeds, and flaxseeds are excellent sources of healthy fats, protein, fiber, and vitamin E. They promote satiety, support blood sugar control, and contribute to brain health.

4. Legumes: Beans, lentils, and chickpeas are a fantastic source of plant-based protein, fiber, B vitamins, and iron. They are a versatile and affordable addition to your diet, promoting gut health and potentially reducing inflammation.

5. Whole Grains: Opt for whole grains like brown rice, quinoa, whole-wheat bread, and oats over refined grains. Whole grains offer sustained energy, fiber, and B vitamins, all crucial for brain function and blood sugar management.

6. Healthy Fats: Avocados, olive oil, and nuts are rich in monounsaturated fats, which promote heart health and may benefit cognitive function. Additionally, healthy fats aid in the absorption of fat-soluble vitamins essential for brain health.

7. Green Tea: This beverage boasts polyphenols, particularly EGCG, an antioxidant with potential neuroprotective properties. Enjoy green tea in moderation, limiting added sugars.

Minimize These Inflammatory Culprits:

1. Added Sugars and Refined Carbohydrates: Sugary drinks, white bread, pastries, and processed foods can cause blood sugar spikes and crashes, potentially impacting mood and cognitive function. They may also contribute to inflammation.

2. Saturated and Trans Fats: Found in processed meats, fried foods, and fatty cuts of red meat, saturated and trans fats can increase inflammation and negatively impact cardiovascular health.

3. Processed Meats: Hot dogs, sausages, bacon, and deli meats are often high in sodium, nitrates, and saturated fat. These can contribute to inflammation and may worsen Parkinson's symptoms.

4. Dairy (Optional): While some research suggests dairy consumption may worsen Parkinson's symptoms in some individuals, it can be a valuable source of calcium and vitamin D. It's best to discuss dairy intake with your doctor or a registered dietitian to determine what's right for you.

Creating a Sustainable and Delicious Eating Pattern:

Creating a sustainable eating pattern that is both brain-boosting and enjoyable is key. Here are some tips:

- ✓ **Focus on Abundance:** Instead of solely focusing on eliminating foods, emphasize incorporating a variety of brain-boosting options into your meals and snacks.
- ✓ **Explore Plant-Based Options:** Explore delicious vegetarian and vegan recipes that incorporate legumes, whole grains, and vegetables for a fiber-rich and nutritious diet.

- ✓ **Spice Up Your Life:** Herbs and spices not only add flavor but also possess anti-inflammatory properties. Experiment with turmeric, ginger, cinnamon, and chili peppers.
- ✓ **Cook More at Home:** This allows you to control ingredients and portion sizes. Make healthy cooking fun by involving family or friends.
- ✓ **Plan Your Meals:** Planning meals and snacks in advance can help you avoid unhealthy choices when pressed for time.
- ✓ **Make Small Changes:** Don't overwhelm yourself with drastic dietary changes. Start by incorporating one or two brain-boosting foods into your daily routine and gradually build from there.

CHAPTER 6:

TIPS FOR EASY MEAL PLANNING WITH PARKINSON'S:

Streamlining Groceries and Meals, Adapting Recipes

Living with Parkinson's can present challenges in the kitchen. This chapter offers practical strategies for simplifying meal planning, grocery shopping, and meal preparation, while ensuring you enjoy delicious and nutritious meals.

Streamlining Grocery Shopping:

- ✓ **Plan Your Meals:** Dedicate some time each week to plan your meals for the upcoming days. Consider including leftovers for lunch or dinner the following day to minimize cooking time.
- ✓ **Make a Grocery List:** Stick to your meal plan when creating your grocery list. This helps avoid impulse purchases and ensures you have everything you need for the week's meals.

- ✓ **Shop Online or with Delivery Services:** Consider online grocery shopping or delivery services to save time and energy. This can be especially helpful if mobility is a challenge.
- ✓ **Shop During Off-Peak Hours:** Avoid crowded stores by shopping during off-peak hours. This can create a calmer and less stressful shopping experience.
- ✓ **Delegate Tasks:** If possible, enlist the help of a family member, friend, or caregiver for grocery shopping. This can make the process easier and more manageable.

Simplifying Meal Preparation:

- ✓ **Prep in Advance:** Dedicate a specific time each week to prepping ingredients for upcoming meals. This could involve washing and chopping vegetables, pre-cooking grains like brown rice or quinoa, or marinating meats.
- ✓ **Utilize Kitchen Tools:** Invest in tools that can make meal prep easier, such as a food processor for chopping vegetables, a slow cooker for hands-off cooking, or single-serving containers for portion control.
- ✓ **Cook Once, Eat Twice:** Cook larger batches of protein sources like chicken or fish and use them in different meals

throughout the week. This saves time and reduces the need for daily cooking.
- ✓ **Freeze Leftovers:** Portion leftovers into single-serving containers and freeze them for quick and easy meals on busy days.
- ✓ **Involve Others:** Cooking can be a social activity! Involve family members or friends in meal preparation to make it more enjoyable and share the workload.

Adapting Recipes for Different Dietary Needs:

- ✓ **Swapping Ingredients:** Many recipes can be easily adapted to accommodate different dietary needs.
- ✓ **For those with swallowing difficulties:** Choose softer cuts of meat, cook vegetables until tender, and consider pureeing soups or stews.
- ✓ **For those with a low-fiber diet:** Opt for peeled fruits and vegetables and limit high-fiber grains like brown rice or whole-wheat bread.
- ✓ **For those on a low-dairy diet:** Use dairy alternatives like unsweetened almond milk or coconut milk in place of dairy milk. Consider calcium-fortified options if needed.
- ✓ **For those with a gluten intolerance:** Choose gluten-free grains like quinoa, brown rice, or certified gluten-free pasta and bread options.

- ✓ **Seasoning is Key:** Even simple dishes can be flavorful with the right spices and herbs. Experiment with different flavor combinations to keep meals interesting.
- ✓ **Focus on Presentation:** Plating your food in an appealing way can make a big difference in how much you enjoy it. Use colorful ingredients, arrange them attractively, and garnish with fresh herbs for a restaurant-worthy feel.

Additional Tips:

- ✓ **Keep a Well-Stocked Pantry:** Having staples like canned beans, whole-grain pasta, dried fruits and nuts, and canned tomatoes on hand allows for quick and easy meal creation.
- ✓ **Embrace Convenience:** Frozen fruits and vegetables are a great option for adding nutrients to meals without the need for chopping or washing. Look for pre-washed and chopped fresh vegetables to save time on prep work.
- ✓ **Don't Be Afraid to Ask for Help:** There are many resources available to help with meal planning and preparation. Consider consulting a registered dietitian for personalized guidance or joining a support group for Parkinson's patients who share meal planning tips.

CHAPTER 7

SAMPLE WEEKLY MEAL PLANS AND GROCERY LISTS:

A Delicious Start to Your Healthy Journey

Planning your meals for the week can be a game-changer, especially when managing Parkinson's. This chapter offers two sample weekly meal plans, complete with breakfast, lunch, dinner, and snack options. Each plan incorporates brain-boosting foods and is accompanied by a corresponding grocery list to streamline your shopping trip.

Sample Weekly Meal Plan 1:

Sunday:

Breakfast (Greek Yogurt Parfait with Berries, Granola, and Honey):

Ingredients:

- 1 cup plain Greek yogurt,

- 1/2 cup mixed berries (blueberries, raspberries, strawberries),
- 1/4 cup granola (low-sugar variety), 1 tablespoon honey (optional)

Instructions:

- In a small parfait glass or bowl, layer 1/3 cup of Greek yogurt, followed by 1/4 cup granola, and 1/3 cup sliced fruit.
- Repeat layers one more time, ending with fruit on top. Drizzle with honey (optional).

Nutritional Facts (per serving):

- Calories: 300, Protein: 15g, Fat: 10g, Carbohydrates: 35g, Fiber: 5g

Tips:

- Use pre-cut frozen fruit for a quick and convenient option. Substitute other nuts like cashews or walnuts for granola. Opt for raw, unsalted nuts for a lower sodium option.

Lunch

(Tuna Salad Sandwich on Whole-Wheat Bread with Lettuce, Tomato, and Avocado Slices, Side Salad with Mixed Greens and Vinaigrette Dressing):

Ingredients:

- 2 slices whole-wheat bread, 1 can (5 oz) tuna packed in water, drained, 1/4 cup mayonnaise (low-fat or light mayonnaise), 1 tablespoon chopped celery (optional), 1 tablespoon chopped red onion (optional), lettuce leaves, tomato slices, 1/2 avocado, sliced, mixed greens, vinaigrette dressing (optional)

Instructions:

- In a bowl, combine tuna, mayonnaise, celery (optional), and red onion (optional). Mash with a fork until desired consistency. Spread tuna salad on one slice of bread, top with lettuce, tomato, and avocado slices. Top with the other slice of bread. Serve with a side salad of mixed greens with vinaigrette dressing (optional).

Nutritional Facts (per serving, including salad with light vinaigrette):

- Calories: 450, Protein: 30g, Fat: 15g, Carbohydrates: 40g, Fiber: 5g

Tips:

Dinner (Salmon with Roasted Vegetables and Quinoa):

Ingredients:

- 2 salmon fillets (6 oz each), 1 tablespoon olive oil, 1 teaspoon dried dill, salt and pepper to taste, 1 cup broccoli florets, 1 cup asparagus spears, 1 red bell pepper, sliced, 1 cup cooked quinoa

Instructions:

- Preheat oven to 400°F (200°C). In a small bowl, combine olive oil and dill.
- Season salmon fillets with salt and pepper. Place salmon on a baking sheet lined with parchment paper.
- Brush salmon with olive oil mixture. Arrange broccoli florets, asparagus spears, and bell pepper slices around the salmon. Roast for 15-20 minutes, or until salmon is cooked through and vegetables are tender-crisp. Serve with cooked quinoa.

Nutritional Facts (per serving):

- Calories: 500, Protein: 40g, Fat: 20g, Carbohydrates: 40g, Fiber: 5g

Tips:

- Substitute cod or another mild white fish for salmon. Use pre-cut vegetables to save time on prep work.
- Cook quinoa according to package instructions.

Snacks:

- Trail mix with nuts, seeds, and dried fruit (see recipe in Chapter 3)
- Apple slices with almond butter (1 apple, 2 tablespoons almond butter)

Sample Weekly Meal Plan 2 (Vegetarian Option):

Sunday:

Breakfast (Chia Pudding with Almond Milk, Berries, and Chia Seeds):

Ingredients:

- 1/2 cup chia seeds
- 1 cup unsweetened almond milk

- 1/2 cup mixed berries (blueberries, raspberries, strawberries)
- 1 tablespoon honey (optional)

Instructions:

- In a small bowl or jar, combine chia seeds, almond milk, and berries. Stir well.
- Refrigerate overnight or for at least 2 hours. In the morning, stir again before serving. Drizzle with honey (optional).

Monday:

Breakfast (Scrambled Eggs with Spinach and Whole-Wheat Toast):

Ingredients:

- 2 eggs, 1 tablespoon olive oil
- 1/2 cup chopped spinach, salt and pepper to taste, 2 slices whole-wheat toast

Instructions

- In a small bowl, whisk together eggs.
- Heat olive oil in a non-stick pan over medium heat.

- Add spinach and cook until wilted.
- Pour in whisked eggs and scramble until cooked through. Season with salt and pepper to taste. Serve scrambled eggs on whole-wheat toast.

Nutritional Facts (per serving):

- Calories: 350, Protein: 20g, Fat: 15g, Carbohydrates: 20g, Fiber: 2g

Tips:

- Add chopped mushrooms, onions, or peppers to the scrambled eggs for additional flavor and nutrients.
- Use a non-stick pan to prevent sticking and reduce the need for added oil.

Lunch

(Leftover Salmon with a Side of Brown Rice and Steamed Green Beans):

Ingredients:

- Leftover salmon from Sunday dinner, cooked brown rice, steamed green beans

Instructions:

- Reheat leftover salmon according to your preference (microwave, oven, stovetop).
- Serve with a side of cooked brown rice and steamed green beans.

Nutritional Facts (per serving, will vary depending on amount of leftover salmon):

- Calories: 400-500, Protein: 30g-40g, Fat: 10g-20g, Carbohydrates: 40g-50Mg, Fiber: 5g

Tips:

- Leftovers can be easily transformed into new meals.
- Flake leftover salmon and toss with a light vinaigrette for a salmon salad on a bed of greens.

Dinner (Chicken Stir-Fry with Brown Rice and Mixed Vegetables):

Ingredients:

- 1 boneless, skinless chicken breast, cut into bite-sized pieces,
- 1 tablespoon soy sauce, 1 tablespoon cornstarch, 1 tablespoon vegetable oil, 1 cup broccoli florets, 1 cup

sliced carrots, 1 red bell pepper, sliced, 1 cup cooked brown rice

Instructions:

- In a bowl, combine chicken pieces, soy sauce, and cornstarch. Marinate for 15 minutes.
- Heat vegetable oil in a large skillet or wok over medium-high heat. Add chicken and cook until browned and cooked through. Add broccoli florets, carrots, and bell pepper slices. Stir-fry for 5-7 minutes, or until vegetables are tender-crisp. Serve stir-fry over cooked brown rice.

Nutritional Facts (per serving):

- Calories: 450, Protein: 35g, Fat: 15g, Carbohydrates: 40g, Fiber: 5g

Tips

- Substitute tofu or tempeh for chicken for a vegetarian option. Add other vegetables of your choice, such as snow peas, snap peas, or baby corn.

Snacks:

- Cottage cheese with sliced peaches (1/2 cup cottage cheese, 1/2 peach, sliced)
- Handful of almonds (approximately 1/4 cup)

Tuesday:

Breakfast (Oatmeal with Chopped Walnuts, Blueberries, and a Sprinkle of Cinnamon):

Ingredients:

- 1/2 cup rolled oats, 1 cup water or milk, 1/4 cup chopped walnuts, 1/4 cup blueberries, 1 teaspoon ground cinnamon

Instructions

- In a saucepan, combine oats and water or milk. Bring to a boil, then reduce heat and simmer for 5-7 minutes, or until oats are cooked through and creamy.
- Stir in chopped walnuts and blueberries. Serve topped with a sprinkle of ground cinnamon.

Nutritional Facts (per serving, made with water):

- Calories: 300, Protein: 5g, Fat: 10g, Carbohydrates: 45g, Fiber: 5g

Tips:

- Use quick oats for a faster cook time.
- For added sweetness, use a drizzle of honey or maple syrup (be mindful of sugar intake).
- Top with other chopped nuts or seeds like chia seeds or flaxseeds for extra nutrients.

Lunch

(Lentil Soup with a Side Salad and Whole-Wheat Bread):

Ingredients:

- Leftover lentil soup from Sunday lunch, side salad with mixed greens and vinaigrette dressing (optional), whole-wheat bread slices

Instructions:

- Reheat leftover lentil soup. Serve with a side salad of mixed greens with vinaigrette dressing (optional) and whole-wheat bread slices.

Nutritional Facts

- (per serving, will vary depending on amount of leftover soup

Dinner

(Turkey Chili with Whole-Wheat Cornbread (optional)):
Ingredients:

For the chili:

- 1 tablespoon olive oil, 1 onion, chopped, 1 green pepper, chopped, 2 cloves garlic, minced, 1 pound ground turkey, 1 (15 oz) can diced tomatoes, undrained, 1 (15 oz) can kidney beans, rinsed and drained, 1 (15 oz) can black beans, rinsed and drained, 1 cup vegetable broth, 1 tablespoon chili powder, 1 teaspoon ground cumin, 1/2 teaspoon dried oregano, salt and pepper to taste
- For the cornbread (optional):
- Follow a pre-made cornbread mix according to package instructions, or use a healthy homemade recipe.

Instructions:

- In a large pot, heat olive oil over medium heat. Add onion and green pepper. Cook for 5 minutes, or until softened. Add garlic and cook for 1 minute more.
- Crumble ground turkey into the pot and cook until browned, breaking it up with a spoon.

- Stir in diced tomatoes, kidney beans, black beans, vegetable broth, chili powder, cumin, oregano, salt, and pepper. Bring to a boil, then reduce heat and simmer for 30 minutes, or until flavors meld.
- Serve chili hot, with your preferred toppings (shredded cheese, chopped onions, sour cream, avocado slices).
- If desired, prepare cornbread according to package instructions or a healthy recipe and serve alongside the chili.

Snacks:

- Edamame pods with a sprinkle of sea salt (1 cup shelled edamame)
- Banana with a dollop of natural peanut butter (1 banana, 2 tablespoons peanut butter)

Wednesday:

Breakfast

(Smoothie made with Greek Yogurt, Berries, Spinach, and a Splash of Almond Milk):

Ingredients:

- 1 cup plain Greek yogurt

- 1/2 cup mixed berries (blueberries, raspberries, strawberries), 1/2 cup fresh spinach, 1/2 cup unsweetened almond milk

Instructions:

- In a blender, combine Greek yogurt, berries, spinach, and almond milk. Blend until smooth and creamy. Serve immediately.
- Nutritional Facts (per serving): Calories: 350, Protein: 20g, Fat: 10g, Carbohydrates: 40g, Fiber: 5g

Tips:

- Use frozen fruit for a thicker consistency and to add coldness to the smoothie. Substitute other greens like kale for spinach.

Lunch (Chickpea Salad Sandwich on Whole-Wheat Bread with Lettuce, Tomato, and Cucumber):

Ingredients:

For the chickpea salad:

- 1 (15 oz) can chickpeas, rinsed and drained, 1/4 cup chopped celery, 1/4 cup chopped red onion, 2 tablespoons mayonnaise (low-fat or light mayonnaise), 1 tablespoon lemon juice, 1/2 teaspoon dried dill, salt and pepper to taste

For the sandwich:

- 2 slices whole-wheat bread, lettuce leaves, tomato slices, cucumber slices

Instructions:

- In a bowl, mash together chickpeas with a fork, leaving some texture. Stir in chopped celery, red onion, mayonnaise, lemon juice, dill, salt, and pepper.
- Spread chickpea salad on one slice of whole-wheat bread. Top with lettuce, tomato slices, and cucumber slices. Top with the other slice of bread.

Nutritional Facts (per serving):

- Calories: 400, Protein: 15g, Fat: 10g, Carbohydrates: 50g, Fiber: 5g

Tips:

- Add other chopped vegetables to the chickpea salad, such as bell peppers or carrots.

- Use a vegan mayonnaise option for a plant-based meal.

Dinner (Baked Cod with Roasted Sweet Potato and Steamed Asparagus):

Ingredients:

- 2 cod fillets (6 oz each),
- 1 tablespoon olive oil
- 1 teaspoon dried oregano, salt and pepper to taste, 1 medium sweet potato, chopped, 1 bunch asparagus, trimmed

Instructions:

- Preheat oven to 400°F (200°C). Lightly grease a baking sheet.
- In a small bowl, combine olive oil and oregano. Season cod fillets with salt and pepper. Place cod fillets on the prepared baking sheet. Brush cod with olive oil mixture.
- Toss chopped sweet potato with a

PART 3: LIVING A VIBRANT LIFE WITH PARKINSON'S:

CHAPTER 8:

ADDITIONAL LIFESTYLE TIPS FOR OPTIMAL HEALTH:

Exercise, Sleep, and Stress Management

Living with Parkinson's requires a multifaceted approach to managing your health. While medication plays a vital role, incorporating healthy lifestyle habits can significantly improve your overall well-being and quality of life. This chapter explores the importance of exercise, sleep, and stress management, along with practical strategies to integrate them into your daily routine.

The Power of Exercise:

Regular physical activity offers a multitude of benefits for people with Parkinson's. It can:

- **Improve motor function and coordination:** Exercise helps maintain muscle strength, flexibility, and balance, which can become increasingly challenging with Parkinson's.

- **Boost mood and energy levels:** Physical activity releases endorphins, natural mood elevators that combat fatigue and depression, common symptoms of Parkinson's.
- **Promote better sleep:** Regular exercise can improve sleep quality, leading to increased energy and a more positive outlook.
- **Slow disease progression:** Studies suggest that exercise may slow the progression of Parkinson's symptoms.

Finding the Right Exercise for You:

There's no one-size-fits-all approach to exercise with Parkinson's. The key is to choose activities you enjoy and can do safely. Here are some excellent options to consider:

- **Walking:** A simple yet effective way to improve cardiovascular health, build endurance, and maintain flexibility. Start with short walks and gradually increase the duration and intensity as tolerated.
- **Swimming:** The buoyancy of water provides low-impact exercise that's easy on the joints, making it a great choice for those with mobility limitations.
- **Tai Chi and Yoga:** These mind-body practices enhance balance, coordination, and flexibility while promoting relaxation and stress reduction.

- **Cycling (stationary or outdoor):** Improves leg strength and cardiovascular health with minimal impact on joints.
- **Strength training:** Building muscle mass can improve balance, coordination, and overall function. Start with light weights and gradually increase intensity under the guidance of a physical therapist or personal trainer experienced in Parkinson's care.

Importance of a Good Night's Sleep:

Sleep is crucial for everyone, but especially for those with Parkinson's. Adequate sleep allows the body to rest, repair, and replenish essential neurotransmitters. When sleep is disrupted, it can worsen Parkinson's symptoms such as tremors, stiffness, and fatigue.

Tips for Better Sleep:

- **Establish a regular sleep schedule:** Go to bed and wake up at the same time each day, even on weekends. Consistency helps regulate your body's natural sleep-wake cycle.
- **Create a relaxing bedtime routine:** Take a warm bath, read a book, or listen to calming music before bed. Avoid

stimulating activities like watching TV or using electronic devices for at least an hour before sleep.

- **Optimize your sleep environment:** Make sure your bedroom is dark, quiet, and cool. Invest in a comfortable mattress and pillows.
- **Limit caffeine and alcohol intake:** Both substances can interfere with sleep quality. Avoid caffeine in the afternoon and evening, and limit alcohol consumption.
- **Regular exercise:** As mentioned earlier, regular physical activity promotes better sleep. However, avoid strenuous exercise close to bedtime.
- **Manage stress:** Stress can disrupt sleep patterns. Relaxation techniques like deep breathing and meditation can help manage stress and improve sleep quality.

Stress Management for Parkinson's:

Chronic stress can exacerbate Parkinson's symptoms and hinder your overall well-being. Learning effective stress management techniques can make a significant difference in your quality of life. Here are some helpful strategies:

Relaxation Techniques:

- **Deep breathing:** Focus on slow, deep breaths from your diaphragm. Breathe in through your nose for a count of four, hold for a count of four, and exhale slowly through your mouth for a count of eight. Repeat for several minutes.

- **Progressive Muscle Relaxation:** Tense and relax different muscle groups throughout your body one at a time. Focus on the feeling of relaxation as you release the tension.
- **Guided Meditation:** There are many guided meditations available online or in apps. These can help you focus on the present moment and quiet your mind.
- **Mindfulness practices:** Mindfulness teaches you to focus on the present moment without judgment. It can help you manage negative thoughts and anxieties that contribute to stress.
- **Connect with others:** Social interaction and support from loved ones can be a powerful stress buffer. Join a support group for people with Parkinson's or connect with friends and family.
- **Seek professional help:** If you're struggling to manage stress on your own, consider talking to a therapist. They can help you develop coping skills and manage stress effectively.

CHAPTER 9

COOKING WITH PARKINSON'S

Helpful Adaptations for Independence in the Kitchen

Living with Parkinson's can present challenges in the kitchen, but with a few adaptations and the right tools, you can continue to enjoy preparing delicious and nutritious meals. This chapter explores kitchen tools and techniques that can simplify meal prep while promoting your independence and safety.

Essential Kitchen Tools for Parkinson's Management:

- **Rocking or Rolling Cutting Boards:** These boards stay put on your countertop, minimizing the risk of slipping or the board sliding while chopping ingredients.
- **Weighted Utensils:** The added weight can improve grip strength and control, making tasks like stirring and mixing easier.
- **Rocker Knife:** This knife features a rocking motion that requires less hand and wrist movement compared to a traditional knife.

- **Jar Openers:** Electric or manual jar openers eliminate the need for excessive twisting and gripping.
- **Adaptive Grippers:** These silicone or rubber grippers provide a better hold on slippery items like pot lids or jars.
- **Peelers with Wide, Easy-Grip Handles:** These make peeling fruits and vegetables less strenuous on your hands.
- **Single-Handed Can Crushers:** These tools allow you to crush cans with minimal effort, reducing the need for two-handed operation.
- **Slow Cooker or Instant Pot:** These appliances offer a convenient and hands-off way to cook healthy meals. Simply add ingredients and let them cook for several hours while you focus on other tasks.
- **Food Processor or Blender:** These appliances can chop, puree, and mix ingredients, saving time and effort.

Kitchen Techniques for Easier Meal Preparation:

- **Prep in Advance:** Dedicate a specific time each week to wash, chop, and pre-cook ingredients for upcoming meals. This minimizes prep work required on cooking days.
- **Utilize Pre-Cut and Pre-Washed Produce:** Many grocery stores offer pre-cut and pre-washed fruits and vegetables, saving you time and effort.

- **Simplify Recipes:** Choose recipes with minimal ingredients and steps. Focus on one-pot meals or sheet pan dinners that require minimal cleanup.
- **Cook in Larger Batches:** Cooking a larger batch of protein like chicken or fish allows for leftovers that can be used in other meals throughout the week. This reduces the need for daily cooking.
- **Embrace Frozen Fruits and Vegetables:** Frozen options are readily available, nutritious, and require no chopping or washing.
- **Thicken Soups and Stews:** Adding thickeners like cornstarch or arrowroot slurry can make soups and stews easier to eat with a spoon.
- **Adapt Utensils:** Use tools like rocker knives, weighted utensils, or utensil grips to improve your grasp and control.

Maintaining Independence in the Kitchen:

- **Organize Your Kitchen:** Keep frequently used items within easy reach and arrange them in a way that promotes efficient movement.
- **Improve Lighting:** Ensure adequate lighting throughout your kitchen workspace to enhance visibility and reduce the risk of accidents.

- **Clear Away Clutter:** Maintain clear countertops and walkways to prevent tripping hazards.
- **Delegate Tasks:** Don't be afraid to ask for help with grocery shopping, carrying heavy items, or cleaning up. This allows you to focus on tasks you can comfortably manage.
- **Modify Your Approach:** If chopping vegetables is challenging, consider using a food processor or pre-cut options. There's no shame in adapting methods to maintain your independence.

Additional Tips:

- **Invest in a Comfortable Chair:** Having a comfortable chair with good back support can make standing for long periods while cooking more manageable.
- **Take Breaks:** Don't try to do too much at once. Schedule breaks throughout your cooking time to avoid fatigue or discomfort.
- **Most Importantly, Have Fun!:** Cooking should be an enjoyable experience. Experiment with new flavors, listen to music, or watch a cooking show while preparing meals.

Remember:

With a little creativity and these helpful adaptations, you can continue to enjoy the satisfaction and health benefits of cooking delicious meals in your own kitchen, regardless of the challenges presented by Parkinson's. Don't hesitate to ask your doctor, occupational therapist, or a kitchen supply store for personalized recommendations on tools and techniques that can best suit your needs.

BONUS
Parkinson's-Friendly Recipes for Beginners:

Delicious and Easy Meals

This section offers easy and delicious recipes incorporating brain-boosting ingredients suitable for a Parkinson's diet. Each recipe highlights the featured ingredients and includes nutritional information and tips for modifications.

Breakfast

Power Berry Oatmeal (Serves 1)

Ingredients:

- 1/2 cup rolled oats
- 1 cup water or milk
- 1/4 cup mixed berries (blueberries, raspberries, strawberries)
- 1/4 cup chopped walnuts
- 1 teaspoon ground cinnamon
- (Optional) 1 tablespoon honey or maple syrup

Instructions:

- In a saucepan, combine oats and water or milk. Bring to a boil, then reduce heat and simmer for 5-7 minutes, or until oats are cooked through and creamy.
- Stir in berries, walnuts, and cinnamon.
- Serve warm. Drizzle with honey or maple syrup (optional).

Nutritional Facts (approx., without added sweetener):

- Calories: 300, Protein: 5g
- Fat: 10g, Carbohydrates: 45g, Fiber: 5g

Tips:

- Use quick oats for a faster cook time.
- Substitute other nuts or seeds like chia seeds or flaxseeds for extra nutrients.

Scrambled Eggs with Spinach and Tomatoes (Serves 1)

Ingredients:

- 2 eggs
- 1 tablespoon olive oil
- 1/2 cup chopped spinach
- 1/4 cup chopped tomato

- Salt and pepper to taste

Instructions:

- In a small bowl, whisk together eggs.
- Heat olive oil in a non-stick pan over medium heat. Add spinach and cook until wilted.
- Pour in whisked eggs and scramble until cooked through.
- Stir in chopped tomatoes. Season with salt and pepper to taste.
- Serve immediately.

Nutritional Facts (approx.):

- Calories: 300,
- Protein: 20g
- Fat: 15g
- Carbohydrates: 5g, Fiber: 1g

Tips:

- Add chopped mushrooms or onions for additional flavor and nutrients. Use a non-stick pan to prevent sticking and reduce the need for added oil.

Greek Yogurt Parfait with Berries and Granola (Serves 1)

Ingredients:

- 1 cup plain Greek yogurt
- 1/2 cup mixed berries (blueberries, raspberries, strawberries)
- 1/4 cup granola (low-sugar variety)
- 1 tablespoon honey (optional)

Instructions:

- In a small parfait glass or bowl, layer 1/3 cup of Greek yogurt, followed by 1/4 cup granola, and 1/3 cup sliced fruit. Repeat layers one more time, ending with fruit on top.
- Drizzle with honey (optional).

Nutritional Facts (approx., without added sweetener):

- Calories: 300, Protein: 15g, Fat: 10g, Carbohydrates: 35g, Fiber: 5g

Tips:

- Use pre-cut frozen fruit for a quick and convenient option. Substitute other nuts like cashews or walnuts for granola. Opt for raw, unsalted nuts for a lower sodium option.

Chia Pudding with Berries and Almond Milk (Serves 1)

Ingredients:

- 1/2 cup chia seeds
- 1 cup unsweetened almond milk
- 1/2 cup mixed berries (blueberries, raspberries, strawberries)
- 1 teaspoon honey (optional)

Instructions:

- In a small bowl or jar, combine chia seeds, almond milk, and berries. Stir well. Refrigerate overnight or for at least 2 hours.
- In the morning, stir again before serving. Drizzle with honey (optional).

Nutritional Facts (approx., without added sweetener):

- Calories: 300, Protein: 5g, Fat: 12g, Carbohydrates: 35g, Fiber: 10g

Tips:

- For a thicker consistency, use a 1:3 ratio of chia seeds to almond milk (1/2 cup chia seeds to 1 1/2 cups almond milk).
- Chia pudding can be stored in the refrigerator for up to 3 days. Experiment with different fruit combinations.

Whole-Wheat Toast with Sliced Avocado and Eggs (Serves 1)

Ingredients:

- 2 slices
- 2 slices whole-wheat toast
- 1/2 avocado, sliced
- 2 hard-boiled eggs, sliced
- Salt and pepper to taste

Instructions:

- Toast whole-wheat bread slices.
- Mash avocado slightly with a fork or keep sliced.
- Arrange avocado slices on toast. Top with sliced hard-boiled eggs.
- Season with salt and pepper to taste.

Nutritional Facts (approx.): Calories:

- 350, Protein: 15g, Fat: 20g, Carbohydrates: 30g, Fiber: 5g

Tips:

- Use a ripe avocado for easier mashing.
- Drizzle with a touch of lemon juice to prevent browning.

Smoothie with Greek Yogurt, Berries, and Spinach (Serves 1)

Ingredients:

- 1 cup plain Greek yogurt
- 1/2 cup mixed berries (blueberries, raspberries, strawberries)
- 1/2 cup fresh spinach
- 1/2 cup unsweetened almond milk

Instructions:

- In a blender, combine Greek yogurt, berries, spinach, and almond milk. Blend until smooth and creamy.
- Serve immediately.

Nutritional Facts (approx.): Calories:

- 350, Protein: 20g
- Fat: 10g, Carbohydrates: 40g, Fiber: 5g

Tips

- Use frozen fruit for a thicker consistency and to add coldness to the smoothie
- Substitute other greens like kale for spinach.

Banana Pancakes with Walnuts (Serves 1)

Ingredients:

- 1 ripe banana, mashed
- 1 egg
- 1/4 cup whole-wheat flour
- 1/4 cup milk (dairy or non-dairy)
- 1/4 teaspoon baking powder
- 1/4 cup chopped walnuts
- Maple syrup (optional)

Instructions:

- In a medium bowl, mash the banana. Whisk in the egg, flour, milk, and baking powder until just combined.
- Heat a lightly greased pan or griddle over medium heat. Pour batter onto the pan, forming small pancakes. Sprinkle some chopped walnuts on top of each pancake.
- Cook for 2-3 minutes per side, or until golden brown.
- Serve warm with a drizzle of maple syrup (optional).

Nutritional Facts (approx., without added sweetener):

- Calories: 350, Protein: 10g, Fat: 15g, Carbohydrates: 45g, Fiber: 5g

Tips:

- Use a non-stick pan to prevent sticking.
- Add a pinch of cinnamon to the batter for extra flavor.

Scrambled Tofu with Vegetables (Serves 1)

Ingredients:

- 1/4 block firm tofu, crumbled
- 1 tablespoon olive oil
- 1/2 cup chopped vegetables (bell peppers, onions, mushrooms)
- 1/4 cup chopped spinach
- Salt and pepper to taste

Instructions:

- In a non-stick pan, heat olive oil over medium heat. Crumble tofu into the pan and cook until slightly golden brown.
- Add chopped vegetables and cook until softened.

- Stir in spinach and cook until wilted.
- Season with salt and pepper to taste.
- Serve scrambled tofu with a whole-wheat toast or whole-grain wrap.

Nutritional Facts (approx.):

- Calories: 250, Protein: 20g, Fat: 10g, Carbohydrates: 20g, Fiber: 2g

Tips:

- Use pre-crumbled tofu for a time-saving option.
- Add a splash of soy sauce or your favorite low-sodium seasoning for additional flavor.

Overnight Oats with Berries and Chia Seeds (Serves 1)

Ingredients:

- 1/2 cup rolled oats
- 1/2 cup milk (dairy or non-dairy)
- 1/4 cup chia seeds
- 1/4 cup mixed berries (blueberries, raspberries, strawberries)
- 1/4 teaspoon ground cinnamon
- (Optional) 1 tablespoon honey or maple syrup

Instructions:

- In a small jar or container, combine oats, milk
- chia seeds, berries, and cinnamon. Stir well. Cover and refrigerate overnight or for at least 2 hours.
- In the morning, stir again before serving. Drizzle with honey or maple syrup (optional).

Nutritional Facts (approx., without added sweetener):

- Calories: 300
- Protein: 5g, Fat: 10g, Carbohydrates: 40g, Fiber: 10g

Tips Use a variety of berries for a flavor and nutritional boost. Add a scoop of nut butter for extra protein and healthy fats.

Cottage Cheese with Sliced Fruit and Honey (Serves 1)

Ingredients:

- 1/2 cup low-fat cottage cheese
- 1/2 cup sliced fruit (apples, pears, peaches)
- 1 tablespoon honey

Instructions:

- In a bowl, combine cottage cheese and sliced fruit.
- Drizzle with honey and stir gently.

Nutritional Facts (approx.):

- Calories: 200, Protein: 15g, Fat: 5g, Carbohydrates: 25g, Fiber: 1g

Tips:

- Use canned fruit in its own juice for a convenient option. Substitute other toppings like chopped nuts or granola for added texture and flavor.

Lunch

Salmon with Roasted Vegetables (Serves 1)

Ingredients:

- 4 oz salmon fillet
- 1 tablespoon olive oil
- 1/2 cup chopped vegetables (broccoli, carrots, asparagus)
- Salt and pepper to taste
- 1/4 cup cooked brown rice

Instructions:

- Preheat oven to 400°F (200°C).

- Toss chopped vegetables with olive oil, salt, and pepper. Spread on a baking sheet.
- Place salmon fillet on top of the vegetables.
- Bake for 15-20 minutes, or until salmon is cooked through and vegetables are tender-crisp.
- Serve salmon with cooked brown rice.

Nutritional Facts (approx.):

- Calories: 450, Protein: 30g, Fat: 20g, Carbohydrates: 35g, Fiber: 5g

Tips:

- Use other fatty fish options like trout or mackerel.
- Marinate the salmon in a mixture of lemon juice, herbs, and spices for additional flavor before baking.

Greek Yogurt Chicken Salad Sandwich (Serves 1)

Ingredients:

- 2 slices whole-wheat bread
- 1/2 cup shredded cooked chicken breast
- 1/4 cup plain Greek yogurt
- 1 tablespoon chopped celery
- 1/4 teaspoon dried dill

- Salt and pepper to taste
- Lettuce or spinach leaves (optional)

Instructions:

- In a bowl, combine shredded chicken, Greek yogurt, chopped celery, dill, salt, and pepper. Mix well.
- Spread chicken salad mixture onto one slice of whole-wheat bread. Top with lettuce or spinach leaves (optional). Add the other slice of bread to create a sandwich.

Nutritional Facts (approx.):

- Calories: 350
- Protein: 30g, Fat: 5g, Carbohydrates: 40g, Fiber: 2g

Tips:

- Use leftover chicken or rotisserie chicken for a quick and easy lunch option.
- Add chopped grapes or cranberries for a touch of sweetness and extra texture.

Tuna Salad with Whole-Wheat Crackers (Serves 1)

Ingredients:

- 1 can (5 oz) canned tuna in water, drained

- 1 tablespoon light mayonnaise
- 1 tablespoon chopped celery
- 1/4 teaspoon dried onion powder
- Salt and pepper to taste
- Whole-wheat crackers

Instructions:

- In a bowl, combine flaked tuna, mayonnaise, chopped celery, onion powder, salt, and pepper. Mix well.
- Serve tuna salad with whole-wheat crackers.

Nutritional Facts (approx.):

- Calories: 300, Protein: 25g, Fat: 10g, Carbohydrates: 25g, Fiber: 2g

Tips:

- Use chopped red onion instead of celery for a different flavor profile.
- Opt for low-fat or fat-free mayonnaise to reduce fat content.

Egg Salad Sandwich with Avocado (Serves 1)

Ingredients:

- 2 slices whole-wheat bread
- 2 hard-boiled eggs, mashed
- 1/4 avocado, mashed
- 1 tablespoon light mayonnaise
- 1 tablespoon chopped onion
- Salt and pepper to taste
- Lettuce or spinach leaves (optional)

Instructions:

- In a bowl, combine mashed eggs, avocado, mayonnaise, chopped onion, salt, and pepper. Mix well.
- Spread egg salad mixture onto one slice of whole-wheat bread. Top with lettuce or spinach leaves (optional). Add the other slice of bread to create a sandwich.

Nutritional Facts (approx.):

- Calories: 400, Protein: 20g, Fat: 20g, Carbohydrates: 30g, Fiber: 5g

Tips:

- Use a ripe avocado for easier mashing.
- Drizzle with a touch of lemon juice to prevent avocado browning. Substitute chopped celery for onion for a different flavor.

Lentil Soup with Whole-Wheat Bread (Serves 1)

Ingredients:

- 1 cup cooked lentils
- 2 cups vegetable broth
- 1/2 cup chopped vegetables (carrots, celery, onions)
- 1 tablespoon olive oil
- 1/2 teaspoon dried thyme
- Salt and pepper to taste

Instructions:

- In a saucepan, heat olive oil over medium heat. Add chopped vegetables and cook until softened.
- Pour in vegetable broth, lentils, and thyme. Bring to a boil, then reduce heat and simmer for 15-20 minutes, or until lentils are tender.
- Season with salt and pepper to taste.

- Serve warm with a slice of whole-wheat bread.

Nutritional Facts (approx.):

- Calories: 350, Protein: 15g, Fat: 10g, Carbohydrates: 45g, Fiber: 10g

Tips:

- Use pre-cooked lentils to save time.
- Add a can of diced tomatoes for extra flavor and lycopene content.

Chicken and Veggie Wrap (Serves 1)

Ingredients:

- 1 large whole-wheat tortilla
- 1/2 cup shredded cooked chicken breast
- 1/4 cup chopped lettuce
- 1/4 cup chopped tomato
- 1/4 cup shredded carrots
- 2 tablespoons hummus

Instructions:

- Spread hummus evenly on a whole-wheat tortilla.

- Arrange shredded chicken, chopped lettuce, tomato, and carrots on top of the hummus.
- Roll the tortilla tightly to create a wrap.

Nutritional Facts (approx.):

- Calories: 400, Protein: 30g, Fat: 10g, Carbohydrates: 40g, Fiber: 5g

Tips:

- Use other lean protein options like grilled fish or tofu.
- Add a sprinkle of chopped fresh herbs for extra flavor.

Berry Salad with Walnuts and Yogurt Dressing (Serves 1)

Ingredients:

- 1 cup mixed berries (blueberries, raspberries, strawberries)
- 1/4 cup chopped walnuts
- 1/4 cup plain Greek yogurt
- 1 tablespoon honey
- 1/4 teaspoon vanilla extract

Instructions:

- In a bowl, combine mixed berries and chopped walnuts.

- In a separate bowl, whisk together Greek yogurt, honey, and vanilla extract.
- Drizzle yogurt dressing over the berry and walnut mixture. Toss gently to coat.

Nutritional Facts (approx.):

- Calories: 300, Protein: 10g, Fat: 15g, Carbohydrates: 35g, Fiber: 5g

Tips:

- Use other fruits like sliced apple or pear for variation.
- Substitute low-fat yogurt for Greek yogurt to reduce fat content.

Open-Faced Turkey and Avocado Sandwich (Serves 1)

Ingredients:

- 1 slice whole-wheat bread
- 1/4 cup sliced turkey breast
- 1/4 avocado, sliced
- 1 tablespoon mashed cottage cheese
- 1 tablespoon chopped tomato
- Lettuce or spinach leaves (optional)

Instructions:

- Toast a slice of whole-wheat bread.
- Spread mashed cottage cheese on the toasted bread.
- Arrange sliced turkey, avocado, and chopped tomato on top of the cottage cheese.
- Add lettuce or spinach leaves (optional).

Nutritional Facts (approx.):

- Calories: 350, Protein: 25g,
- Fat: 15g, Carbohydrates: 30g, Fiber: 3g

Tips:

- Use leftover turkey or deli-sliced turkey for a quick and easy option.
- Drizzle with a balsamic vinegar reduction for a flavorful twist.

Cottage Cheese with Fruit and Granola (Serves 1)

Ingredients:

- 1/2 cup low-fat cottage cheese
- 1/2 cup chopped fruit (apples, pears, peaches)
- 1/4 cup granola (low-sugar variety)

Instructions:

- In a bowl, combine cottage cheese, chopped fruit, and granola.
- Stir gently to combine.

Nutritional Facts (approx.):

- Calories: 300, Protein: 15g, Fat: 5g,
- Carbohydrates: 40g, Fiber: 5g

Tips:

- Use a variety of fruits for added flavor and nutrients.
- Substitute chopped nuts or seeds for granola for a different texture.

Egg Salad Lettuce Wraps (Serves 1)

Ingredients:

- 2 large lettuce leaves
- 2 hard-boiled eggs, mashed
- 1 tablespoon light mayonnaise
- 1 tablespoon chopped celery
- 1/4 teaspoon dried dill
- Salt and pepper to taste

Instructions:

- In a bowl, combine mashed eggs, mayonnaise, chopped celery, dill, salt, and pepper. Mix well.
- Wash and dry large lettuce leaves.
- Spoon egg salad mixture onto each lettuce leaf.
- Roll up the lettuce leaves to create wraps.

Nutritional Facts (approx.):

- Calories: 250, Protein: 15g,
- Fat: 10g, Carbohydrates: 5g, Fiber: 1g

Tips:

- Use romaine lettuce or butter lettuce leaves for sturdy wraps.
- Add a sprinkle of chopped fresh herbs like chives or parsley for extra flavor.

Dinner

Baked Salmon with Roasted Vegetables and Quinoa (Serves 1)
Ingredients:

- 4 oz salmon fillet
- 1 tablespoon olive oil
- 1/2 cup chopped vegetables (broccoli, carrots, asparagus)
- 1/4 cup cooked quinoa
- Salt and pepper to taste
- Lemon wedges (optional)

Instructions:

- Preheat oven to 400°F (200°C).
- Toss chopped vegetables with olive oil, salt, and pepper. Spread on a baking sheet.
- Place salmon fillet on top of the vegetables.
- Bake for 15-20 minutes, or until salmon is cooked through and vegetables are tender-crisp.
- Serve salmon with cooked quinoa. Garnish with lemon wedges (optional).

Nutritional Facts (approx.):

- Calories: 500, Protein: 35g,
- Fat: 25g, Carbohydrates: 40g, Fiber: 5g

Tips

- Use other fatty fish options like trout or mackerel.

- Marinate the salmon in a mixture of lemon juice, herbs, and spices for additional flavor before baking.

Scrambled Eggs with Spinach, Tomatoes, and Whole-Wheat Toast (Serves 1)

Ingredients:

- 2 eggs
- 1 tablespoon olive oil
- 1/2 cup chopped spinach
- 1/4 cup chopped tomatoes
- 2 slices whole-wheat bread
- Salt and pepper to taste

Instructions:

- In a non-stick pan, heat olive oil over medium heat.
- Add chopped spinach and cook until wilted.
- Add chopped tomatoes and cook for another minute.
- Whisk eggs in a bowl and pour into the pan with the vegetables. Scramble until cooked through.
- Toast whole-wheat bread slices.
- Serve scrambled eggs on top of toast. Season with salt and pepper to taste.

Nutritional Facts (approx.):

- Calories: 400, Protein: 25g, Fat: 15g, Carbohydrates: 35g, Fiber: 5g

Tips:

- Add crumbled feta cheese or shredded mozzarella for extra protein and flavor.
- Use a non-stick pan to prevent sticking.

Greek Yogurt Chicken Bowl with Berries (Serves 1)

Ingredients:

- 1/2 cup cooked shredded chicken breast
- 1/2 cup plain Greek yogurt
- 1/4 cup mixed berries (blueberries, raspberries, strawberries)
- 1/4 cup chopped walnuts
- 1/4 cup chopped vegetables (cucumber, bell peppers)
- 1 tablespoon olive oil
- Salt and pepper to taste

Instructions:

- In a bowl, combine cooked shredded chicken, Greek yogurt, and salt and pepper to taste. Mix well.
- Arrange chopped vegetables and berries on the side of the bowl.
- Drizzle with olive oil and sprinkle with chopped walnuts.

Nutritional Facts (approx.)

- Calories: 400, Protein: 30g,
- Fat: 15g, Carbohydrates: 30g, Fiber: 5g

Tips

- Use leftover chicken or rotisserie chicken for a quick and easy option.
- Substitute other fruits like sliced apple or pear for berries.

Turkey Meatloaf with Roasted Vegetables (Serves 1)

Ingredients:

- 1/2 pound lean ground turkey
- 1/4 cup chopped onion
- 1/4 cup chopped mushrooms
- 1/4 cup chopped bell peppers
- 1/4 cup breadcrumbs
- 1 egg, beaten

- 1 tablespoon olive oil
- 1/2 cup chopped vegetables (broccoli, carrots)
- Salt and pepper to taste

Instructions:

- Preheat oven to 375°F (190°C).
- In a bowl, combine ground turkey, chopped onion, mushrooms, bell peppers, breadcrumbs, egg, salt, and pepper. Mix well.
- Form the mixture into a loaf shape and place in a baking dish.
- Toss chopped vegetables with olive oil and spread around the meatloaf.
- Bake for 30-35 minutes, or until the meatloaf is cooked through and vegetables are tender.

Nutritional Facts (approx.):

- Calories: 450, Protein: 40g
- Fat: 20g, Carbohydrates: 30g, Fiber: 5g

Tips:

- Use a meat thermometer to ensure the internal temperature of the meatloaf reaches 165°F (74°C) for safe consumption.

- Substitute ground chicken or lean beef for ground turkey.

Whole-Wheat Pasta with Shrimp and Vegetables (Serves 1)

Ingredients:

- 1/2 cup cooked whole-wheat pasta
- 4 oz shrimp, peeled and deveined
- 1 tablespoon olive oil
- 1/2 cup chopped vegetables (broccoli, carrots, zucchini)
- 1/4 cup chopped cherry tomatoes
- 1/4 cup low-sodium vegetable broth
- 1 tablespoon chopped fresh parsley
- Salt and pepper to taste

Instructions:

- Cook whole-wheat pasta according to package instructions.
- In a pan, heat olive oil over medium heat. Add shrimp and cook until pink and opaque, about 2-3 minutes per side.
- Add chopped vegetables and cook until tender-crisp.
- Pour in vegetable broth and simmer for a minute.
- Toss in cooked pasta and chopped parsley. Season with salt and pepper to taste.

Nutritional Facts (approx.):

- Calories: 400, Protein: 30g,
- Fat: 10g, Carbohydrates: 45g, Fiber: 5g

Tips:

- Use frozen pre-cooked shrimp for a time-saving option.
- Substitute other vegetables like asparagus or bell peppers for variation.

Walnut-Crusted Salmon with Roasted Brussels Sprouts (Serves 1)

Ingredients:

- 4 oz salmon fillet
- 1/4 cup chopped walnuts
- 1 tablespoon olive oil
- 1/2 cup Brussels sprouts, trimmed and halved
- Salt and pepper to taste
- Lemon wedges (optional)

Instructions:

- Preheat oven to 400°F (200°C).
- In a food processor, pulse chopped walnuts until coarsely ground.

- Coat salmon fillet with olive oil, salt, and pepper. Press the ground walnuts onto the salmon to create a crust.
- Toss Brussels sprouts with olive oil, salt, and pepper. Spread on a baking sheet.
- Place the salmon fillet on top of the Brussels sprouts.
- Bake for 15-20 minutes, or until salmon is cooked through and Brussels sprouts are tender-crisp.
- Serve with lemon wedges (optional).

Nutritional Facts (approx.):

- Calories: 500, Protein: 35g
- Fat: 30g, Carbohydrates: 20g, Fiber: 5g

Tips:

- Use a mixture of chopped walnuts and breadcrumbs for the crust. Substitute other vegetables like broccoli florets or cauliflower florets for Brussels sprouts.

Egg Drop Soup with Vegetables (Serves 1)

Ingredients:

- 2 cups low-sodium chicken broth
- 1 egg, beaten

- 1 tablespoon cornstarch mixed with 2 tablespoons water (cornstarch slurry)
- 1/4 cup chopped vegetables (mushrooms, spinach, carrots)
- 1 tablespoon soy sauce (low-sodium)
- Salt and pepper to taste

Instructions:

- In a saucepan, bring chicken broth to a simmer.
- Slowly drizzle in the beaten egg while stirring constantly to create egg ribbons.
- Stir in the cornstarch slurry and cook for a minute until the soup thickens slightly.
- Add chopped vegetables and soy sauce. Simmer for another minute.
- Season with salt and pepper to taste.

Nutritional Facts (approx.):

- Calories: 200, Protein: 10g, Fat: 5g,
- Carbohydrates: 20g, Fiber: 1g

Tips:

- Use vegetable broth instead of chicken broth for a vegan option. Add a sprinkle of chopped green onions for extra flavor.

Cottage Cheese with Fruit and Granola

(This recipe is similar to breakfast #9, but can be enjoyed for dinner as well)

Ingredients:

- 1/2 cup low-fat cottage cheese
- 1/2 cup chopped fruit (apples, pears, peaches)
- 1/4 cup granola (low-sugar variety)

Instructions:

- In a bowl, combine cottage cheese, chopped fruit, and granola. Stir gently to combine.

Nutritional Facts (approx.):

- Calories: 300, Protein: 15g, Fat: 5g, Carbohydrates: 40g, Fiber: 5g

Tips:

- Use a variety of fruits for added flavor and nutrients.

- Substitute chopped nuts or seeds for granola for a different texture.

Snacks

Fruit and Nut Mix (Serves 1)

Ingredients:

- 1/2 cup mixed berries (blueberries, raspberries, strawberries)
- 1/4 cup chopped walnuts
- 1 tablespoon dried cranberries

Instructions:

- In a bowl, combine berries, chopped walnuts, and dried cranberries.

Nutritional Facts (approx.):

- Calories: 300, Protein: 5g, Fat: 15g, Carbohydrates: 30g, Fiber: 5g

Tips:

- Use a variety of fruits and nuts for added flavor and nutrients. Substitute other dried fruits like chopped dates or apricots for cranberries.

Greek Yogurt with Chia Seeds and Honey (Serves 1)

Ingredients:

- 1/2 cup plain Greek yogurt
- 1 tablespoon chia seeds
- 1 teaspoon honey

Instructions:

- In a bowl, combine Greek yogurt, chia seeds, and honey. Stir well.
- Refrigerate for at least 15 minutes to allow the chia seeds to absorb the yogurt and thicken the mixture.

Nutritional Facts (approx.):

- Calories: 150, Protein: 10g, Fat: 5g, Carbohydrates: 15g, Fiber: 3g

Tips:

- Use flavored Greek yogurt for a variation in taste. Substitute maple syrup or agave nectar for honey.

Hard-Boiled Eggs with Sliced Vegetables (Serves 1)

Ingredients:

- 2 hard-boiled eggs
- 1/2 cup sliced vegetables (cucumber, carrots, bell peppers)
- Hummus (optional)

Instructions:

- Peel the hard-boiled eggs and slice them into halves or quarters.
- Wash and slice vegetables into sticks or bite-sized pieces.

Nutritional Facts (approx.):

- Calories: 200, Protein: 12g, Fat: 5g, Carbohydrates: 5g, Fiber: 2g

Tips:

- Prepare a batch of hard-boiled eggs at the beginning of the week for a convenient grab-and-go snack. Serve with hummus for added protein and healthy fats.

Trail Mix (Serves 1)

Ingredients:

- 1/4 cup unsalted almonds
- 1/4 cup dried raisins
- 1/4 cup pumpkin seeds
- 1 tablespoon dark chocolate chips (optional)

Instructions:

- In a small container or bag, combine almonds, raisins, pumpkin seeds, and dark chocolate chips (optional).

Nutritional Facts (approx.):

- Calories: 300, Protein: 5g, Fat: 15g, Carbohydrates: 30g, Fiber: 5g

Tips:

- Adjust the ingredients based on your preferences. Substitute other nuts, seeds, or dried fruits for variety. Choose dark chocolate with a high cacao content for added antioxidants.

Cottage Cheese with Pineapple and Sliced Almonds (Serves 1)

Ingredients:

- 1/2 cup low-fat cottage cheese
- 1/4 cup chopped pineapple

- 1 tablespoon sliced almonds

Instructions:

- In a bowl, combine cottage cheese, chopped pineapple, and sliced almonds.

Nutritional Facts (approx.):

- Calories: 200, Protein: 15g, Fat: 5g, Carbohydrates: 20g, Fiber: 1g

Tips:

- Use canned pineapple in its own juice for convenience. Substitute other fruits like berries or peaches for pineapple.

Edamame Pods with Sea Salt (Serves 1)

Ingredients:

- 1 cup frozen shelled edamame
- 1/2 teaspoon sea salt

Instructions:

- Cook the frozen edamame according to package instructions (usually boiling or microwaving).
- Drain the edamame and sprinkle with sea salt.

Nutritional Facts (approx.)

- Calories: 180, Protein: 17g, Fat: 8g, Carbohydrates: 10g, Fiber: 5g

Tips

- Look for pre-cooked and shelled edamame for an even quicker snack option.
- Season with other spices like chili powder or garlic powder for added flavor.

Apple Slices with Almond Butter (Serves 1)

Ingredients:

- 1 apple, sliced
- 2 tablespoons almond butter

Instructions:

- Wash and slice the apple.
- Spread almond butter on apple slices.

Nutritional Facts (approx.):

- Calories: 250, Protein: 5g, Fat: 10g, Carbohydrates: 30g, Fiber: 5g

Tips:

- Choose a variety of apple types like Granny Smith for tartness or Fuji for sweetness.
- Substitute other nut butters like peanut butter or cashew butter for almond butter.

Whole-Wheat Crackers with Hummus and Vegetables (Serves 1)

Ingredients:

- 4 whole-wheat crackers
- 1/4 cup hummus
- 1/4 cup sliced vegetables (cucumber, bell peppers, carrots)

Instructions:

- Spread hummus on whole-wheat crackers.
- Arrange sliced vegetables on top of the hummus.

Nutritional Facts (approx.)

- Calories: 250, Protein: 5g, Fat: 10g, Carbohydrates: 30g, Fiber: 5g

Tips:

- Look for low-fat or reduced-sodium hummus options. Experiment with different flavored hummus varieties like roasted red pepper or olive tapenade.

Cottage Cheese Smoothie (Serves 1)

Ingredients:

- 1/2 cup low-fat cottage cheese
- 1/2 cup berries (frozen or fresh)
- 1/4 cup unsweetened almond milk
- 1 tablespoon honey (optional)

Instructions:

- Blend all ingredients together in a blender until smooth.
- Add a little more almond milk if needed to achieve desired consistency.

Nutritional Facts (approx.)

- Calories: 200, Protein: 15g, Fat: 5g, Carbohydrates: 25g, Fiber: 2g

Tips:

- Use a variety of berries for flavor variation.

- Substitute Greek yogurt for cottage cheese for a thicker smoothie consistency.
- Add a sprinkle of spinach or kale for a hidden veggie boost.

Roasted Chickpeas with Spices (Serves 1)

Ingredients:

- 1 can (15 oz) chickpeas, drained and rinsed
- 1 tablespoon olive oil
- 1/2 teaspoon ground cumin
- 1/4 teaspoon chili powder
- 1/4 teaspoon paprika
- Salt and pepper to taste

Instructions:

- Preheat oven to 400°F (200°C).
- Pat the chickpeas dry with a paper towel.
- In a bowl, toss chickpeas with olive oil, cumin, chili powder, paprika, salt, and pepper.
- Spread chickpeas on a baking sheet in a single layer.
- Roast for 20-25 minutes, or until golden brown and crispy.

Nutritional Facts (approx.):

- Calories: 200, Protein: 8g, Fat: 5g, Carbohydrates: 25g, Fiber: 5g

Tips

- Experiment with different spice combinations like garlic powder, onion powder, or smoked paprika.
- Roast the chickpeas with chopped vegetables like broccoli florets or cauliflower florets for added flavor and nutrients.

CONCLUSION

EMBRACING DELICIOUS AND NUTRITIOUS EATING WITH PARKINSON'S DISEASE

Congratulations on taking a proactive step towards your well-being! This Parkinson's-friendly recipe collection has equipped you with 75 easy and delicious meals and snacks that can nourish your body and support your health journey.

As you explored these recipes, you've likely noticed a focus on incorporating key ingredients that can benefit those living with Parkinson's disease. Here's a quick recap:

- ✓ **Fatty Fish:** Rich in omega-3 fatty acids, these fish can play a role in reducing inflammation and potentially improving cognitive function.
- ✓ **Fruits and Vegetables:** Packed with vitamins, minerals, and antioxidants, these offer a multitude of health benefits and can help combat free radical damage.

- ✓ **Whole Grains:** Choosing whole grains over refined carbohydrates provides sustained energy, keeps you feeling fuller for longer, and offers valuable fiber.
- ✓ **Nuts and Seeds:** Excellent sources of healthy fats, protein, and fiber, these can contribute to a sense of satiety and provide essential nutrients.
- ✓ **Greek Yogurt:** A protein powerhouse, Greek yogurt offers a creamy and versatile base for meals and snacks, promoting muscle health and aiding in feeling full.
- ✓ **Personalize your Plate:** Don't be afraid to adjust recipes to suit your preferences and dietary needs. Substitute ingredients, explore different spices, and discover flavor combinations you enjoy.
- ✓ **Focus on Variety:** Incorporate a wide range of fruits, vegetables, whole grains, and protein sources into your meals. This ensures your body receives a spectrum of essential nutrients.
- ✓ **Plan and Prep:** Dedicate some time each week to planning meals and prepping ingredients. This can save time and prevent unhealthy choices when hunger strikes.
- ✓ **Cook Together:** Invite friends and family to join you in the kitchen. Cooking can be a fun and social activity, fostering connection and enjoyment of healthy meals.

- ✓ **Mindful Eating:** Slow down and savor your food. Pay attention to hunger and fullness cues to avoid overeating.
- ✓ **Stay Hydrated:** Drinking plenty of water throughout the day is crucial for overall health and can aid in digestion.
- ✓ Living with Parkinson's disease doesn't have to mean sacrificing flavor or enjoyment when it comes to food. With a little planning and creativity, you can create delicious and nourishing meals that support your health and well-being. We encourage you to continue exploring new recipes, experiment with flavors, and embrace the power of food as you navigate your Parkinson's journey.

Wishing you continued health and happiness!

www.ingramcontent.com/pod-product-compliance
Lightning Source LLC
Chambersburg PA
CBHW050257230526
45471CB00005B/1918